EX - LIB

£4=00

12

LC.26

ACUPUNCTURE ATLAS AND REFERENCE BOOK

A definitive set of charts based on a careful study of most of the known charts and an assessment of each point through over twenty years of practice, designed for quick and easy reference by students and practitioners.

By the same author
    THE ACUPUNCTURE TREATMENT OF MUSCULO-SKELETAL
  CONDITIONS
THE CELESTIAL STEMS
THE NON-MERIDIAL POINTS OF ACUPUNCTURE
THE PRINCIPLES AND PRACTICE OF MOXIBUSTION
  (co-authored with Roger Newman Turner)
THE SECONDARY VESSELS OF ACUPUNCTURE

ACUPUNCTURE ATLAS AND REFERENCE BOOK

by

Royston Low
Ph.D., N.D., D.O., M.B.N.O.A., F.B.Ac.A., DrAc.

Illustrated by
Stephen Lee

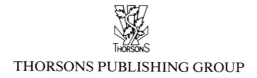

THORSONS PUBLISHING GROUP

First published 1985
This edition first published 1988

To those many students whose
bewilderment prompted me to
attempt a little clarification.

FØ15.89

British Library Cataloguing in Publication Data

Low, Royston, H.

Acupuncture atlas and reference book
1. Acupuncture points — Atlases
I. Title
615.8'92   RM184

ISBN 0-7225-1805-6

*Published by Thorsons Publishers Limited,
Wellingborough, Northamptonshire, NN8 2RQ, England*

Printed in Great Britain by
Woolnough Bookbinding Limited, Irthlingborough, Northamptonshire

1 3 5 7 9 10 8 6 4 2

CONTENTS

INTRODUCTION

Students and practitioners are often bemused by the discrepancies between acupuncture charts issuing from various sources — even the charts from Beijing, Shanghai and Hong Kong differ slightly in the positions given for certain of the points, whilst there are sometimes differences between the charts and written descriptions from the same source.

In an attempt to rectify this situation I have produced what I hope will be considered a definitive set, based on a careful study of most of the known charts and an assessment of each point through over twenty years of practice.

It takes many years of experience before a practitioner can go immediately to any point on the body with unfailing precision, and even then there are always moments of temporary aberration where the exact location just 'slips the memory'.

These charts are designed for quick and easy reference. The student will already have been taught how to locate the points, so I have not bothered with written descriptions, neither have I put in too much extraneous detail. In so far as the extra-meridial points are concerned I assume that practitioners who know enough of their indications to consider their application will already know where they are, and as their inclusion would tend to further 'clutter up' the charts they have been purposely omitted.

It is assumed that all needles are inserted perpendicularly to the skin. Where they need to be inserted at a specific angle this is stipulated in the notes, which also contain details of any special facts about the individual points.

At the end are included all the usual mementos of acupuncture which it is so useful to have at one's finger tips — Five-Element details, Xi-Cleft points and so on, and it is hoped this will make the busy practitioner's life just that little bit more easy.

For details of the internal pathways and re-union points the practitioner should consult the author's book *The Secondary Vessels of Acupuncture*.

LOCATING THE POINTS

Details of the general anatomical measurements are given in all books on acupuncture, but little is written about the best and quickest way to locate the approximate position of the points in a working situation — I say approximate because no system of measurements will ever locate the points exactly; their true position being found only by palpation and experience.

The usual methods given in all the text-books are based upon the length of the middle phalange of the patient's middle fingers, or else the widths of the practitioner's fingers, etc.

My own personal preference is to rely purely upon anatomical landmarks and to look for easily divisible measurements which can be split into equal fractions by the outstretched fingers. The easiest example would be the distance between the sterno-xyphoid junction (CV16) and the umbilicus (CV8), which is 8 cun. Splitting this into half would locate CV12 and also Ki19 and St21 on the same level. Splitting the upper half, between CV12 and 16, gives us CV14 and the levels of Ki21, St19 and (roughly) Li14. Splitting the lower half, between CV12 and CV8, would give us CV10, Ki17 and St23, and each of these halves can be further split for CV9 and CV11, and the appropriate points on their level. The distance between the umbilicus (CV8) and the pubic symphysis is 5 cun, which is difficult to split precisely, so in this case one has to estimate 1/5th up, for CV3, and then split the remaining 4 cun for the other points.

Measurements for the points on the lower leg are all taken on the external aspect — centre of patella to tip of lateral malleolus = 16 cun. Therefore halfway gives us St40, also St38, BL57 and Li8. Halfway between this and the malleolus, i.e. 4 cun up, is GB38 and Sp6. Other points can be found by halving and halving again. The process can be extended to the whole of the body, with the exception of such points as lie in definite hollows etc., such as Co15, TH14, SI10, Lu2, GB34. GB30 is a third of the way between the tip of the great trochanter and the sacro-coccygeal junction.

With an accurate knowledge of the relationship of points on the same level and the necessary landmarks the whole process can be extremely quick and very definite.

ANTERIOR ARM

Lu1	Mu pt of Lu
Lu5	Ho pt — Water pt — Dispersal pt
Lu6	Xi-Cleft pt
Lu7	Lo pt — Key pt of Ren Mai (to affect thumb, slope to thumb; to affect meridian, slope to Lu8)
Lu8	Metal pt — Horary pt
Lu9	Earth pt — Source pt — Tonification pt — Influential pt for vessels
Lu10	Fire pt
Lu11	Wood pt (oblique upwards, 0.1 cun)
Ht3	Ho pt — Water pt
Ht4	Metal pt
Ht5	Lo pt
Ht6	Xi-Cleft pt
Ht7	Earth pt — Source pt — Dispersal pt (either perpendicular *or* oblique to Ht8)
Ht8	Fire pt — Horary pt
Ht9	Wood pt — Tonification pt (oblique upwards, 0.1 cun)
HC1	Oblique 0.2 cun (avoid needling too deeply)
HC3	Ho pt — Water pt
HC4	Xi-Cleft pt
HC5	Metal pt
HC6	Lo pt — Key pt of Yin Wei
HC7	Earth pt — Source pt — Dispersal pt
HC8	Fire pt — Horary pt
HC9	Wood pt — Tonification pt (oblique upwards 0.1 cun)

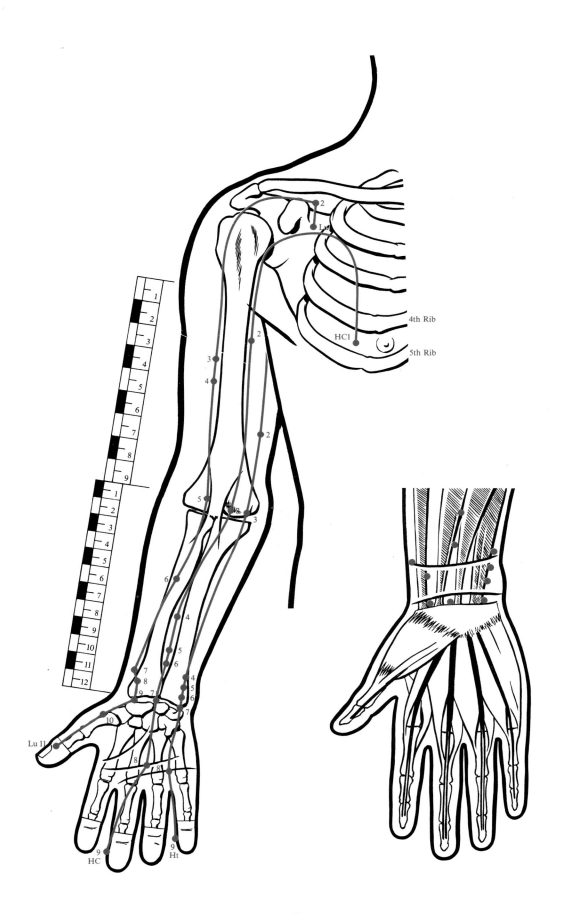

4th Rib

HC1

5th Rib

Lu 11

HC

Ht

POSTERIOR ARM

Co1	Metal pt — Horary pt (oblique upwards 0.1 cun)
Co2	Water pt — Dispersal pt
Co3	Wood pt
Co4	Source pt (direct towards HC8, 0.5-0.8 cun)
Co5	Fire pt
Co6	Lo pt
Co7	Xi-Cleft pt
Co11	Ho pt — Earth pt — Tonification pt
Co13	Moxa only
Co15	Oblique downwards, 0.6-1.2 cun
TH1	Metal pt (oblique upwards, 0.1 cun)
TH2	Water pt (oblique to TH4, 0.3-0.5 cun)
TH3	Wood pt — Tonification pt
TH4	Source pt
TH5	Lo pt — Key pt of Yang Wei
TH6	Fire pt — Horary pt
TH7	Xi-Cleft pt
TH10	Ho pt — Earth pt — Dispersal pt
SI1	Metal pt (oblique upwards, 0.1 cun)
SI2	Water pt
SI3	Wood pt — Tonification pt — Key pt of Du Mai
SI4	Source pt
SI5	Fire pt — Horary pt
SI6	Xi-Cleft pt
SI7	Lo pt
SI8	Ho pt — Earth pt — Dispersal pt
SI11	Obliquely, 0.5-1.0 cun
SI14	Obliquely, 0.3-0.6 cun
SI15	Obliquely, 0.3-0.6 cun

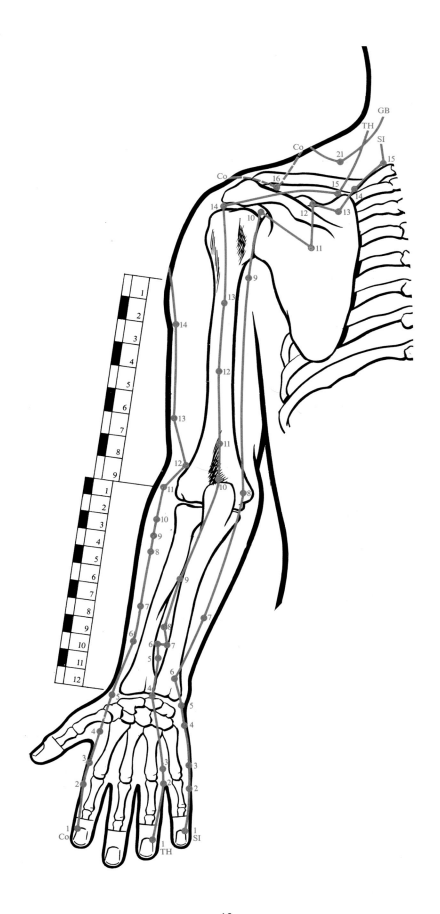

POSTERO-LATERAL ARM

Co1	Metal pt — Horary pt (oblique upwards, 0.1 cun)
Co2	Water pt — Dispersal pt
Co3	Wood pt
Co4	Source pt (direct towards HC8, 0.5-0.8 cun)
Co5	Fire pt
Co6	Lo pt
Co7	Xi-Cleft pt
Co11	Ho pt — Earth pt — Tonification pt
Co13	Moxa only
Co15	Oblique downwards, 0.6-1.2 cun
TH1	Metal pt (oblique upwards, 0.1 cun)
TH2	Water pt (oblique to TH4, 0.3-0.5 cun)
TH3	Wood pt — Tonification pt
TH4	Source pt
TH5	Lo pt — Key pt of Yang Wei
TH6	Fire pt — Horary pt
TH7	Xi-Cleft pt
TH10	Ho pt — Earth pt — Dispersal pt
GB22	Meeting pt of Tendino-Muscular meridians of Shou Yin Lines

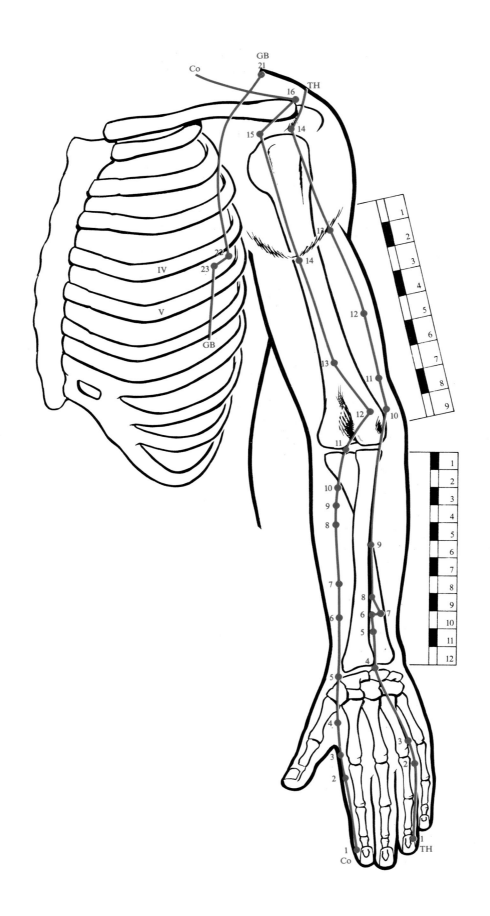

ANTERIOR LEG

St34	Xi-Cleft pt
St35	Needle with knee flexed to right-angle, oblique to Li8, 0.7-1.0 cun
St36	Ho pt
St37	Lower Ho pt of Co
St39	Lower Ho pt of SI
St40	Lo pt
St41	Fire pt — Tonification pt
Sp5	Metal pt — Dispersal pt
Sp6	Union of Tsu Yin lines (contra-indicated during pregnancy)
Sp8	Xi-Cleft pt
Sp9	Ho pt — Water pt
Sp11	0.3-0.5 cun only (deep needling contra-indicated)
Li4	Metal pt
Li5	Lo pt (0.3-0.5 cun horizontally, posteriorly under skin)
Li6	Xi-Cleft pt (0.3-0.5 cun horizontally, posteriorly under skin)
Li12	Moxa only, with roll, 3-5 minutes
GB34	Ho pt — Earth pt — Influential pt for tendons

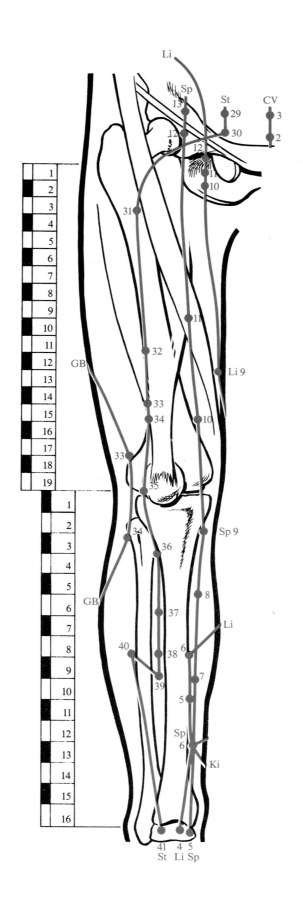

POSTERIOR LEG

Note: The numbering for the Bladder Meridian is the European system.

Bl53	Lower Ho pt of TH
Bl54	Ho pt — Earth pt
Bl58	Lo pt
Bl59	Xi-Cleft pt of Yang Chiao
Bl60	Fire pt (oblique to tip of medial malleolus)

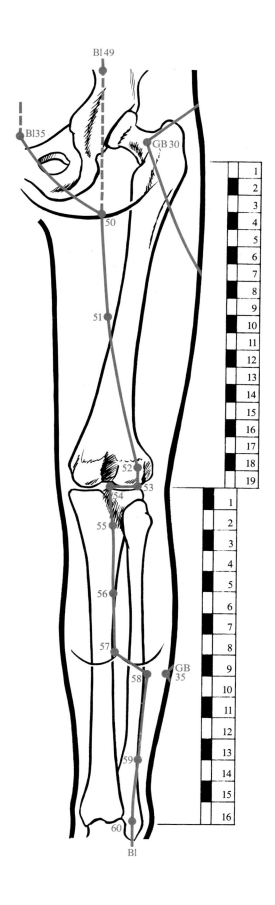

LATERAL LEG

Bl58	Lo pt
Bl59	Xi-Cleft pt of Yang Chiao
Bl60	Fire pt (oblique to tip of medial malleolus)
Bl62	Key pt of Yang Chiao
GB34	Ho pt — Earth pt
GB35	Xi-Cleft pt of Yang Wei
GB36	Xi-Cleft pt of GB
GB37	Lo pt
GB38	Fire pt — Pt of dispersal
GB40	Source pt (slope to Ki3)
St34	Xi-Cleft pt
St35	Oblique to Li8, 0.7-1.0 cun
St36	Ho pt — Earth pt — Horary pt
St37	Lower Ho pt of Co
St39	Lower Ho pt of SI
St40	Lo pt
St41	Fire pt — Tonification pt

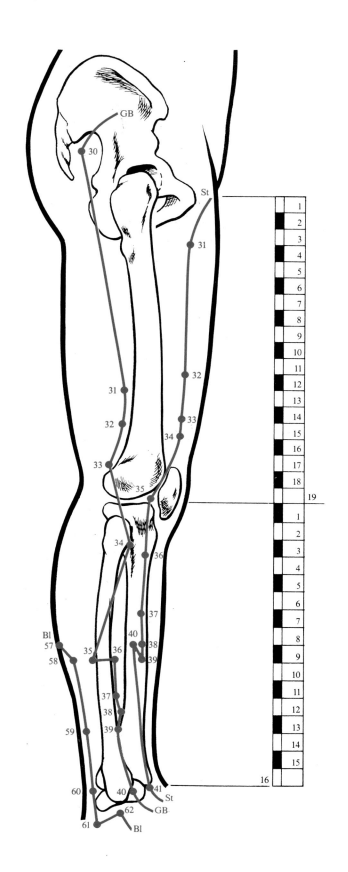

MEDIAL LEG

Sp5	Metal pt — Dispersal pt
Sp6	Union of Tsu Yin lines (contra-indicated during pregnancy)
Sp8	Xi-Cleft pt
Sp9	Ho pt — Water pt
Sp11	0.3-0.5 cun only (deep needling contra-indicated)
Ki3	Source pt — Earth pt (slope to tip of lateral malleolus)
Ki4	Lo pt
Ki5	Xi-Cleft pt
Ki6	Key pt of Yin Chiao
Ki7	Metal pt — Tonification pt
Ki8	Xi-Cleft pt of Yin Chiao
Ki9	Xi-Cleft pt of Yin Wei
Ki10	Ho pt — Water pt — Horary pt
Li4	Metal pt
Li5	Lo pt (horizontally posteriorly under skin, 0.3-0.5 cun)
Li6	Xi-Cleft pt (horizontally posteriorly under skin, 0.3-0.5 cun)
Li8	Ho pt — Water pt — Tonification pt

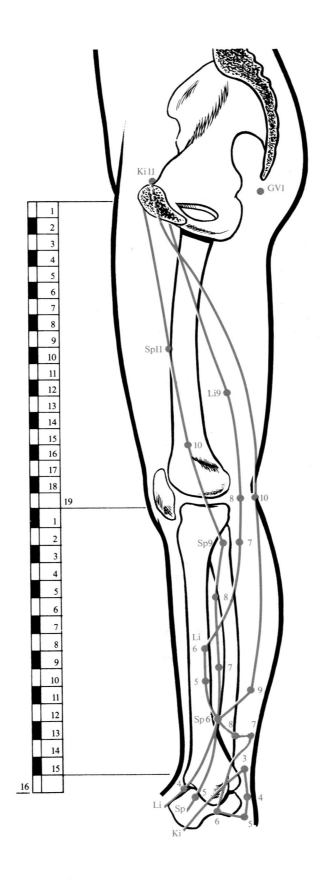

FOOT

Bl58	Lo pt
Bl59	Xi-Cleft pt of Yang Chiao
Bl60	Fire pt (oblique to tip of medial malleolus)
Bl62	Key pt of Yang Chiao
Bl63	Xi-Cleft pt
Bl64	Source pt
Bl65	Wood pt — Dispersal pt
Bl66	Water pt — Horary pt
Bl67	Metal pt — Tonification pt (oblique upwards 0.1 cun)
St39	Lower Ho pt of SI
St40	Lo pt
St41	Fire pt — Tonification pt
St42	Source pt (avoid artery)
St43	Wood pt
St44	Water pt
St45	Metal pt — Dispersal pt (oblique upwards 0.1 cun)
GB35	Xi-Cleft pt of Yang Wei
GB36	Xi-Cleft pt of GB
GB37	Lo pt
GB38	Fire pt — Dispersal pt
GB39	Influential pt of Marrow
GB40	Source pt
GB41	Wood pt — Horary pt — Key pt of Dai Mai
GB43	Water pt — Tonification pt (oblique upwards 0.2-0.3 cun)
GB44	Metal pt (oblique upwards 0.1-0.2 cun)
Sp1	Wood pt (oblique upwards 0.1 cun)
Sp2	Fire pt — Tonification pt
Sp3	Earth pt — Source pt — Horary pt
Sp4	Lo pt — Key pt of Chong Mai
Sp5	Metal pt — Dispersal pt
Sp6	Union of Tsu Yin lines (contra-indicated during pregnancy)
Ki1	Wood pt — Dispersal pt
Ki2	Fire pt
Ki3	Earth pt — Source pt (slope to tip of lateral malleolus)
Ki4	Lo pt
Ki5	Xi-Cleft pt
Ki6	Key pt of Yin Chiao
Ki7	Metal pt — Tonification pt
Ki8	Xi-Cleft pt of Yin Chiao
Ki9	Xi-Cleft pt of Yin Wei

Li1	Wood pt — Horary pt (oblique upwards, 0.1-0.2 cun)
Li2	Fire pt — Dispersal pt (oblique to under hallux, 0.5 cun)
Li3	Earth pt — Source pt (slope to Ki1)
Li4	Metal pt
Li5	Lo pt (horizontally posteriorly, 0.3-0.5 cun)
Li6	Xi-Cleft pt (horizontally posteriorly, 0.3-0.5 cun)

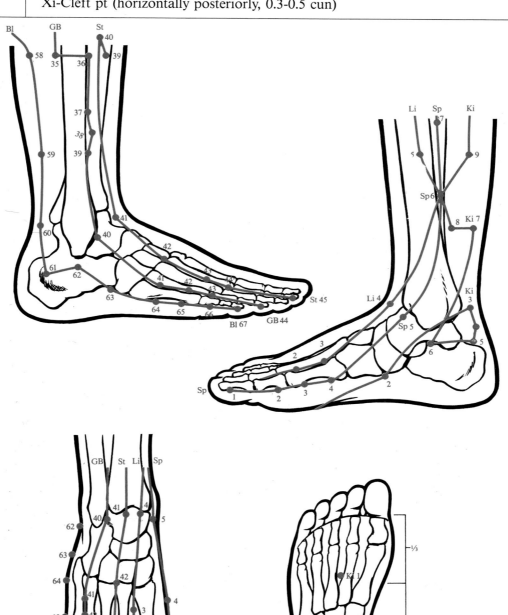

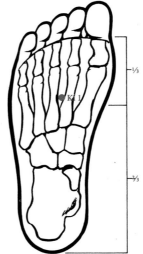

ANTERIOR TRUNK

Lu1 Lu5	Mu pt of Lu Water pt — Ho pt — Dispersal pt
HC1 HC3	Oblique 0.2 cun (avoid needling deeply) Ho pt — Water pt
Ht3	Ho pt — Water pt
St9 St12 St14 ⎫ St15 ⎬ St16 ⎭ St17 St18 St25	Avoid artery Union with Co, TH, GB, SI, T/M of Lu (avoid artery and too deep needling, 0.3-0.5 cun) Oblique 0.3 cun Contra-indicated Oblique 0.3 cun Mu pt of Co
Sp17 Sp18 ⎫ Sp19 ⎬ Sp20 ⎭	Oblique 0.3-0.5 cun
Li12 Li13 Li14	Moxa only (with roll, 3-5 minutes) Mu pt of Sp — Influential pt of Tsang organs Mu pt of Li (oblique 0.3 cun)
Ki22 ⎫ Ki23 ⎪ Ki24 ⎬ Ki25 ⎪ Ki26 ⎭	Oblique 0.3-0.5 cun
CV4 CV5 CV8 CV9 CV12 CV14 CV15 CV16 CV17 CV18 ⎫ CV19 ⎬ CV20 ⎭ CV22	Mu pt of SI Mu pt of TH Moxa only (usually on salt. Can use stick) Special pt for fluid retention Mu pt of St — Influential pt for Fu organs Mu pt of Ht Lo pt of Ren Mai Horizontally along skin, 0.3-0.5 cun Mu pt of HC — Influential pt for Ch'i (horizontally along skin, 0.3-0.5 cun) Horizontally along skin, 0.3-0.5 cun Oblique down behind sternum, 0.5-0.7 cun (not too deep)

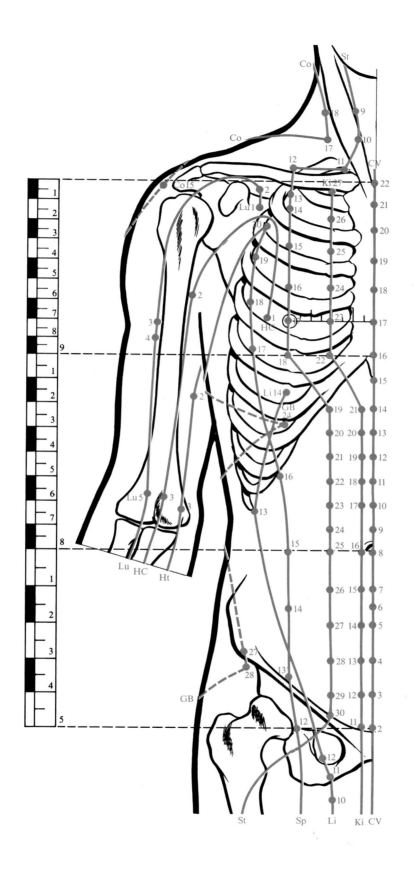

POSTERIOR TRUNK

Co11 Co13 Co15	Earth pt — Tonification pt Moxa only, with roll, 5-10 minutes Oblique downwards, 0.6-1.2 cun
TH10	Ho pt — Earth pt — Dispersal pt
SI8 SI11 SI14 SI15	Ho pt — Earth pt — Dispersal pt Oblique 0.5-1.0 cun Oblique 0.3-0.6 cun Oblique 0.3-0.6 cun
Note: The numbering for the Bl meridian is the European system.	
Bl12-21 inc. Bl22-35 inc. Bl36-45 inc. Bl11 Bl13 Bl14 Bl15 Bl16 Bl17 Bl18 Bl19 Bl20 Bl21 Bl22 Bl23 Bl25 Bl27 Bl28	Either perpendicularly 0.6-1.0 cun, or obliquely 0.6 cun towards spinal column Perpendicularly Oblique downwards, 0.5 cun Influential pt for Bone Back-Shu pt of Lu Back-Shu pt of HC Back-Shu pt of Ht Back-Shu pt of GV Influential pt for Blood Back-Shu pt of Li Back-Shu pt of GB Back-Shu pt of Sp Back-Shu pt of St Back-Shu pt of TH Back-Shu pt of Ki Back-Shu pt of Co Back-Shu pt of SI Back-Shu pt of Bl
GV2 GV9 GV14 GV15	Oblique upwards, 0.5 cun Oblique upwards, 0.5-1.0 cun Meeting pt of Yang meridians Carefully, 0.5-1.0 cun (not too deeply)

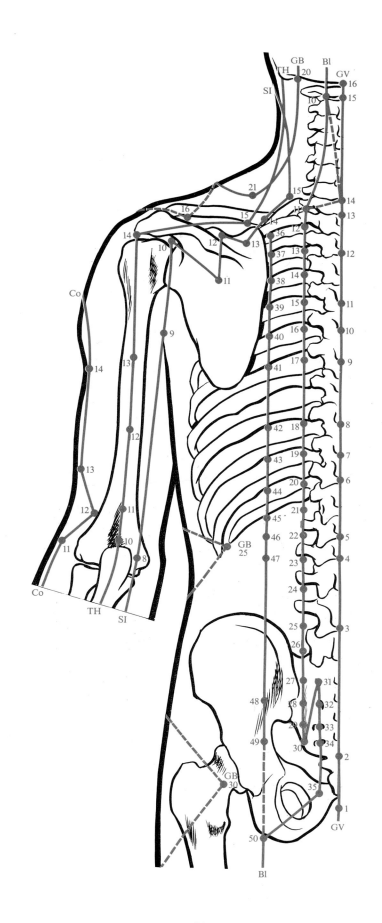

LATERAL TRUNK

GB22	Union of T/Ms of Shou Yin lines
GB23	Oblique 0.3-0.5 cun
GB24	Mu pt of GB (oblique 0.3-0.5 cun)
GB25	Mu pt of Ki
Sp17 Sp18 Sp19 Sp20 Sp21	Oblique 0.3-0.5 cun
St14 St15 St16	Oblique 0.3 cun
St17	Contra-indicated
St18	Oblique 0.3 cun
St25	Mu pt of Co
Li13	Mu pt of Sp — Influential pt of Tsang organs
Li14	Mu pt of Li (oblique 0.3 cun)
Ki22 Ki23 Ki24 Ki25 Ki26	Oblique 0.3-0.5 cun
CV4	Mu pt of SI
CV5	Mu pt of TH
CV8	Moxa only (usually on salt. Can use stick)
CV9	Special pt for fluid retention
CV12	Mu pt of St — Influential pt for Fu organs
CV14	Mu pt of Ht
CV15	Lo pt of Ren Mai
CV16	Horizontally along skin, 0.3-0.5 cun
CV17	Mu pt of HC — Influential pt for Ch'i (horizontally along skin, 0.3-0.5 cun)
CV18 CV19 CV20	Horizontally along skin, 0.3-0.5 cun
CV22	Oblique down behind sternum, 0.5-0.7 cun (not too deep)

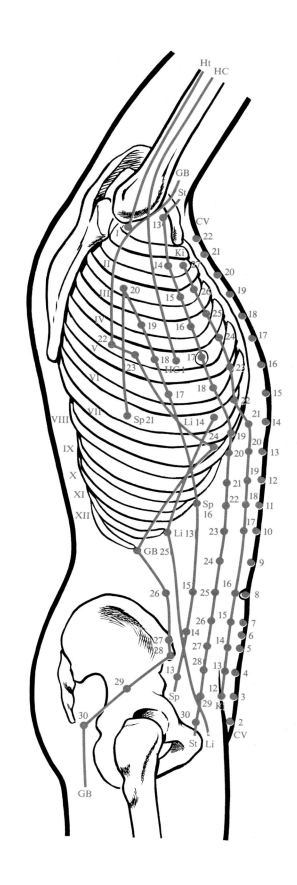

LATERAL HEAD

Co19	Oblique 0.2-0.3 cun
Co20	Obliquely, either downwards 0.3 cun, or towards Bl1
St1	Perpendicularly, along infra-orbital ridge, 0.3-0.7 cun **(NO MOXA)**
St2	Perpendicularly 0.3-0.5 cun, or down to St3 **(NO MOXA)**
St4	Oblique to St6
St5	Oblique to St6
St6	Oblique to St4, or perpendicularly
St8	Horizontally to TH23
St9	Perpendicularly 0.3-0.5 cun (avoid artery)
St12	Perpendicularly 0.3-0.5 cun (not too deep) (union of GB, TH, Co, SI, T/M of Lu)
SI19	Locate with mouth open
TH17	Oblique to internal canthus of opposite eye, with mouth open
TH18	Oblique 0.1 cun, or bleed
TH19	Oblique 0.1 cun
TH20	Oblique downwards 0.1 cun
TH22	Oblique 0.1-0.3 cun (avoid artery)
TH23	Horizontally posteriorly, 0.3 cun
GB1	Horizontally laterally, 0.2-0.3 cun
GB2	Locate with mouth open
GB4 to GB11 inc.	Horizontally posteriorly under skin, 0.2-0.4 cun
GB12	Obliquely downwards, 0.3-0.5 cun
GB13	Horizontally posteriorly, 0.3-0.5 cun
GB14	Horizontally downwards, 0.3-0.5 cun
GB15	Horizontally upwards, 0.3-0.5 cun
GB16 } GB17 } GB18 }	Horizontally posteriorly, 0.3-0.5 cun
GB19	Horizontally downwards, 0.3-0.5 cun
GB20	Perpendicularly to tip of nose, 0.5-1.0 cun
Bl1	Perpendicularly along orbital wall, 0.3 cun, with eyes closed **(NO MOXA)**
Bl2	Horizontally inferiorly or laterally 0.3-0.5 cun, or bleed **(NO MOXA)**
Bl3	Horizontally upwards, 0.3-0.5 cun
Bl4	Horizontally upwards, 0.3-0.5 cun
Bl5-9 inc.	Horizontally 0.3-0.5 cun
GV17-23 inc.	Horizontally 0.3-0.5 cun
GV24	Horizontally upwards, 0.3-0.5 cun
GV25	Perpendicularly, 0.2-0.3 cun
GV26	Oblique upwards, 0.2-0.3 cun

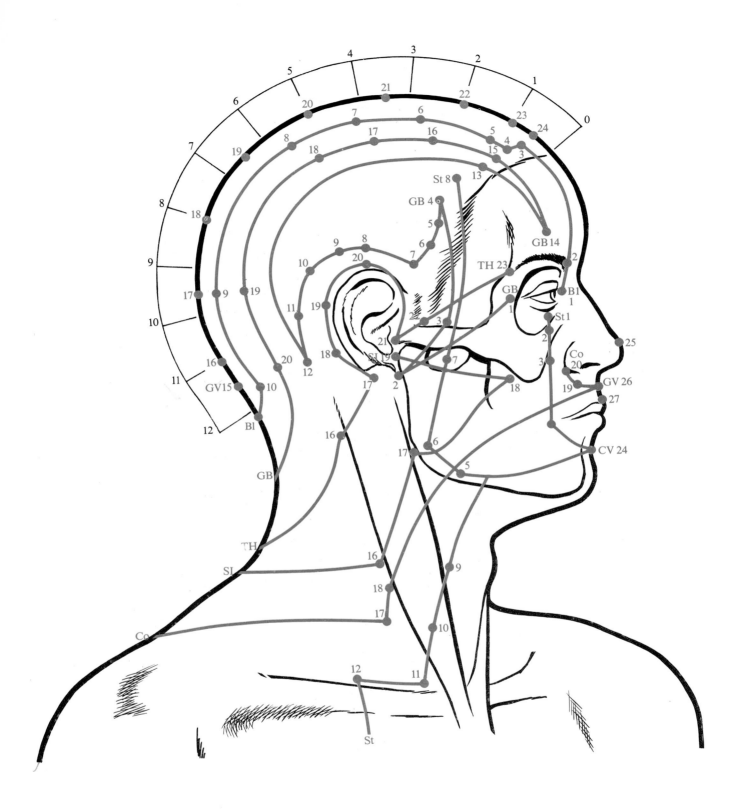

33

FACE

Co19 Co20	Oblique 0.2-0.3 cun Obliquely either downwards or to Bl1, 0.3 cun
St1 St2 St4 St5 St6 St8 St9 St12	Perpendicularly along infra-orbital ridge, 0.3-0.7 cun (**NO MOXA**) Perpendicularly, or down to St3, 0.2-0.3 cun (**NO MOXA**) Oblique to St6 Oblique to St6 Oblique to St4, or perpendicularly Horizontally to TH23 Perpendicularly 0.3-0.5 cun (avoid artery) Perpendicularly 0.3-0.5 cun (not too deep) (union of GB, TH, Co, SI, T/M of Lu)
TH23	Horizontally posteriorly, 0.3 cun
GB1 GB13 GB14 GB15 GB16	Horizontally laterally, 0.2-0.3 cun Horizontally posteriorly, 0.3-0.5 cun Horizontally downwards, 0.3-0.5 cun Horizontally upwards, 0.3-0.5 cun Horizontally posteriorly, 0.3-0.5 cun
Bl1 Bl2 Bl3 Bl4 Bl5	Perpendicularly along orbital wall, 0.3 cun with eyes closed (**NO MOXA**) Horizontally inferiorly or laterally, 0.3-0.5 cun, or bleed (**NO MOXA**) Horizontally upwards, 0.3-0.5 cun Horizontally upwards, 0.3-0.5 cun Horizontally upwards, 0.3-0.5 cun
GV22 GV23 GV24 GV25 GV26 GV27 GV28	Horizontally posteriorly, 0.3-0.5 cun Horizontally upwards, 0.3-0.5 cun Horizontally upwards, 0.3-0.5 cun Perpendicularly, 0.2-0.3 cun Oblique upwards, 0.2-0.3 cun Perpendicularly, 0.2-0.3 cun Oblique upwards, 0.1-0.2 cun, or bleed
CV22 CV23 CV24	Oblique down behind sternum, 0.5-0.7 cun (not too deep) Perpendicularly upwards, 0.5-1.0 cun Oblique upwards, 0.2-0.3 cun

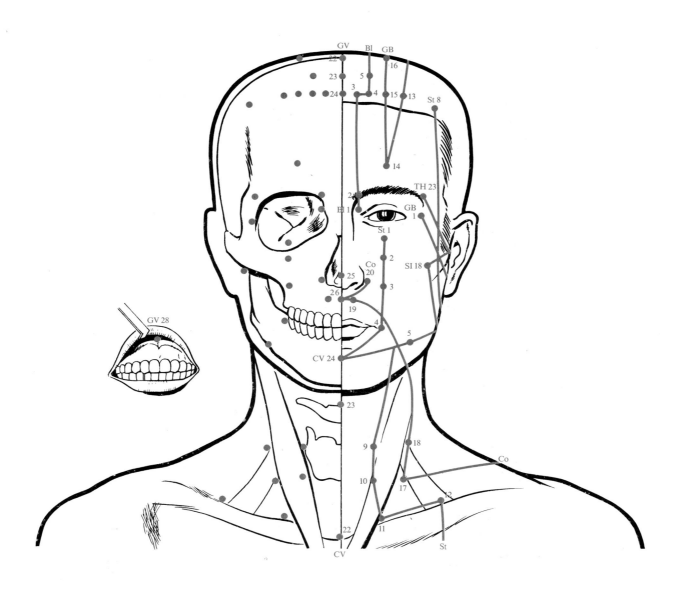

EAR POINTS

Name	No.	Grid Ref.	Name	No.	Grid Ref.
Abdomen	36	Df	Eye (New pt)	90	Ci
Abdomen (Upper)	130	Bj	Eye 1	102	Bk
Abdomen (Lower)	129	Bi	Eye 2	103	Bl
Abdomen (Outside)	37	Ef	Finger	22	Db
Adrenal Gland	93	Bj	Forehead	16	Ck
Ankle Joint	45	Cc			
Anus	113	Bg	Great Yang (Temple)	17	Ck
Apex	18	Dk	Heart	79	Ci
Appendix	67	Ch	Heat pt	38	De
Appendix pt	28	Ej	Heel	44	Cc
Ascites pt	77	Cg	Helix 1	121	Fb
Asthma	12	Cj	Helix 2	122	Gf
Asthma pt	56	Bd	Helix 3	123	Fh
Bladder	70	Ch	Helix 4	124	Fj
Blind Pile pt	115	Bc	Helix 5	125	Em
Brain pt (Pituitary)	14	Dj	Helix 6	126	Cn
Brain Stem	107	Dj	Hepatitis Area	89	Dh
Bronchiectasis	84	Ci	Hepatitis pt	59	Bd
Bronchus	82	Ci,Cj	Hepatomegalia Area	87	Dh
Buttock	49	De	High Blood Pressure	98	Bk
Cardia	63	Ch	Hip Joint	47	Dd
Cardiac pt	106	Bh	Hunger pt	97	Bj
Cheek Area	9	Dm	Inner Ear	7	Dm
Cirrhosis Area	86	Dh	Inner Nose	91	Bj
Clavicle	21	Ej	Internal Secretion	100	Bk
Constipation pt	58	Be	Jowl (Upper)	4	Dl
Dermis (Sub-Cortex)	19	Ck	Jowl (Lower)	5	Dk
Diaphragm	68	Ch	Kidney	71	Cf
Drunk pt	78	Cf	Knee	46	Dd
Dumb Gate	131	Bi	Knee Joint	48	Dc
Duodenum	64	Dh	Large Intestine	66	Bg
Ear Apex	114	Cb	Liver	74	Dg
Ear Centre	69	Ch	Liver Yang 1	119	Eb
Ear (Inner)	7	Dm	Liver Yang 2	120	Fc
Ear (Outer)	105	Bh	Lower Jowl	5	Dk
Elbow	25	Ff	Lowering Pressure	55	Bc
Excitement pt	20	Ck	Lumbago	42	De
External Genitalia	110	Ae	Lumbar Vertebrae	33	Eg
Eye	6	Cm			

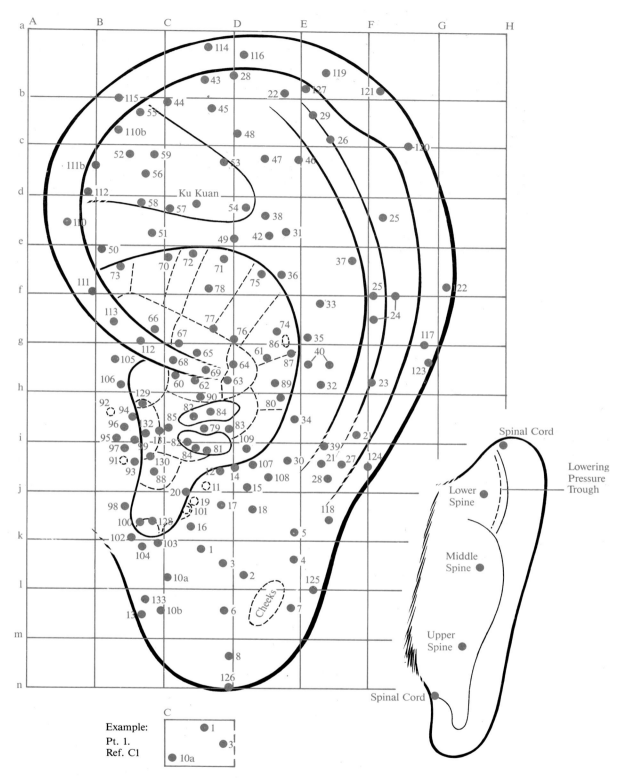

Example:
Pt. 1.
Ref. C1

(Take left-side and lower lines)

Name	No.	Grid Ref.	Name	No.	Grid Ref.
Lung	81	Cj	Small Intestine	65	Ch
			Soft Palate	108	Dj
Mammary Gland	40	Eh	Spleen	80	Di
Minor Occipital Nerve	127	Eb	Stomach	61	Dh
Mouth	60	Ch	Sub-Cortex (Dermis)	19	Ck
			Suprarenal	93	Bj
Neck	34	Di	Sympathetic	50	Bf
Neck Vertebrae	30	Dj			
Nephritis pt	27	Ej	Temple (Gt Yang)	17	Ck
Nerve pt	132	Bi	Testicle (& Ovary)	13	Bm
Neurasthenia pt	133	Bm	Thigh Joint	57	Ce
Nose (Inner)	91	Bj	Thirst pt	96	Bi
Nose (Outer)	95	Bi	Thoracic Vertebrae	32	Eh
Nose-Ear Purification	99	Bj	Thorax	35	Eg
			Throat	92	Bi
Occiput	15	Dj	Thyroid Gland	39	Ej
Oesophagus	62	Ch	Thyroid Gland (2)	128	Bk
Outside Abdomen	37	Ef	Toe	43	Cb
Outer Ear	105	Bh	Tongue	3	Cl
Outer Nose	95	Bi	Tonsil	8	Cn
Ovary	101	Ck	Tonsil (1)	116	Db
Ovary (& Testicle)	13	Bm	Tonsil (2)	117	Fh
			Tonsil (3)	118	Ek
Palate (Upper)	2	Dl	Toothache pt	109	Dj
Palate (Lower)	1	Cl	Tooth Extraction pts	10	Cl,Bm
Pancreas-Gall	75	Df	Trachea	85	Ci
Pancreatitis pt	76	Dg	Tragus Apex	94	Bi
Parotid Gland	11	Cj	Triple Heater	88	Bj
Pelvis Cavum	54	De	Tubercle pt	83	Ci
Pituitary	14	Dj			
Prostate	73	Bf	Upper Jowl	4	Dl
			Ureter	72	Cf
Rectum (Lower section)	112	Bg	Urethra	111	Af
Rising Pressure pt	104	Bl	Urethra (2)	111b	Ad
			Urticaria pt	29	Ec
Sacral Vertebrae	31	De	Uterus	52	Bd
Sciatic Nerve	51	Be			
Shenmen	53	Cd	Wrist	26	Ec
Shoulder	24	Fg			
Shoulder Joint	23	Fh			

NOGIER EAR-POINTS

Name	No.	Ref.	Name	No.	Ref.
Musculo-Skeletal			Maxillary	42	Di
Thumb	1	Cb	Tooth-Extraction (1)	47	Ak
Index Finger	2	Cb	Tooth-Extraction (2)	51	Aj
Middle Finger	3	Cb	*General*		
Third Finger	4	Db	Aggressive pt	49	Ak
Little Finger	5	Dc	Allergy pt	38	Ca
Wrist	6	Ed	Diminishing Libido	39	Dh
Radius	7	Ee	Exciting Libido pt	63	Bf
Ulnar	8	Ee	(Glans Penis & Clitoris)		
Elbow	9	Ef	Headache	48	Ak
Clavicle	10	Eg	Joy pt	45	Ck
Shoulder	11	Eg	'Marvellous pt'		
Scapula	12	Dh	(5th D vertebra)	78	Dh
Atlas	13	Ci	Omega pt	50	Aj
7th Cervical	14	Dg	Sleeping pt	53	Bi
5th Dorsal	15	Df	Sneezing pt	46	Ck
6th Dorsal	81	Cg	Vitality pt (Cancer)	62	Bg
1st Lumbar	16	Ce	*Organs & Tissues*		
5th Lumbar	17	Be	Adenoids	90	Bg
Coccyx	18	Ad	Anus	67	Ad
Breast	19	Df	Bladder	86	Cf
Sternum & Rib area	20	De	Colon — Left	68	Be
Abdominal Muscles	21	Dd	Colon — Left	69	Be
Hallux Toe	22	Cb	Colon — Left	70	Be
Second Toe	23	Bb	Colon — Right	71	Ce
Third Toe	24	Bb	Duodenum	75	Cf
Fourth Toe	25	Bc	Gall-Bladder	72	Cf
Fifth Toe	26	Bc	Genital pt	52	Bi
Heel	27	Bc	Heart (3-4 D vertebrae)	79	Dh
Internal Malleolus	28	Bc	Ileum	73	Ch
External Malleolus	29	Bc	Jejunum	74	Cf
Knee	30	Cc	Kidney	88	Be
Sciatic pt	31	Bd	Labia majora/Scrotum	66	Ae
Sacro-Iliac	32	Cd	Labia minora/Prepuce	65	Be
Buttocks	33	Cd	Larynx	93	Bg
Scarpa's Triangle	34	Cd	Liver	84	Cf
Pubic Symphysis	35	Cd	Mammary Gland	60	Bh
Hip Joint	36	Cd	Mucous Membranes	95	Bh
Coxalgia pt	37	Eb	Pancreas	85	Cf
Temporo-maxillary	40	Di	Skin	96	Bg
Mandible	41	Di			

Name	No.	Ref.
Stomach	76	Dg
Tongue	92	Bg
Tonsils	91	Bg
Ureter	87	Be
Urethra	64	Bf
Uterus	94	Bh
Endocrine & Nervous System		
Adrenal	59	Ai
Anterior Pituitary	54	Bi
Hypogastric plexus (2)	80	Cg
Hypothalamus	55	Bi
Inferior Cervical Gang	77	Dg
Metabolic Regulation pt	44	Dj
Parathyroid	56	Bi
Sensorial pt	43	Cj
Splanchnic Nerve	83	Cg
Solar Plexus	82	Cg
Thermo-Regulation pt	61	Bh
Thymus	58	Bi
Thyroid	57	Bi

Note:

Lobule = Conditioned Reflexes
Root of Helix = Emotions
Tragus = Body Tissues
Antihelix = Spinal Column

A = Cranial Area
B = Intellect Area
C = Olfactory Area
D = Auditory Area
E = Visual Area

Z = Point Zero

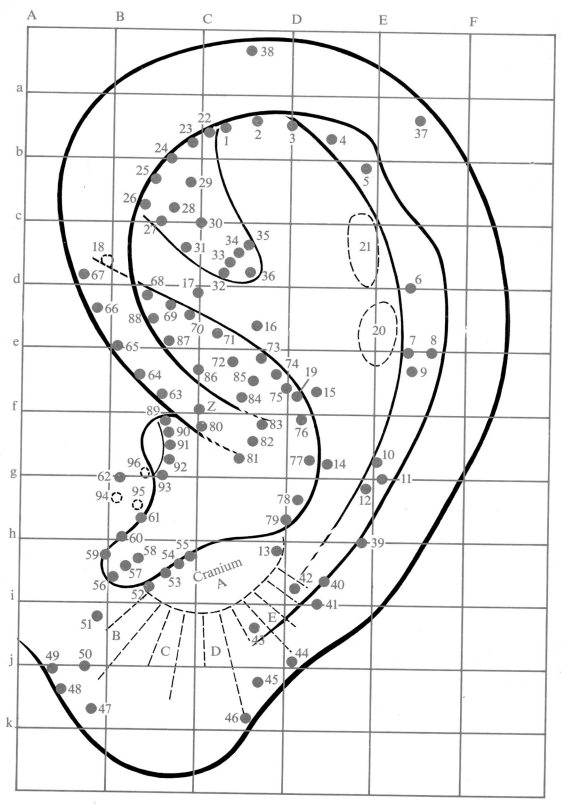

Z = Zero Point

REFERENCE SECTION

Meridian	Back-Shu point	Level of:	Front-Mu point	Xi-Cleft (Accumulation) point	Root	Branch
Lu	Bl13	D3/4	Lu1	Lu6	Lu9	Lu1
Co	Bl25	L4/5	St25	Co7	Co11	Co20
St	Bl21	D12/L1	CV12	St34	St45	St4
Sp	Bl20	D11/12	Li13	Sp8	Sp6	CV23
Ht	Bl15	D5/6	CV14	Ht6	Ht7	Bl15
SI	Bl27	S1	CV4	SI6	SI6	Bl2
Bl	Bl28	S2	CV3	Bl63	Bl59	Bl1
Ki	Bl23	L2/3	GB25	Ki5	Ki6	Bl23
HC	Bl14	D4/5	CV17	HC4	HC6	HC1
TH	Bl22	L1/2	CV5	TH7	TH3	TH23
GB	Bl19	D10/11	GB24	GB36	GB43	GB2
Li	Bl18	D9/10	Li14	Li6	Li4	Bl18

The Irregular (Eight Extra) Vessels:

Vessel	Points	Key point
Du Mai	Own specific points (Lo pt GV1)	SI3
Yang Chiao Mai	Bl62, Bl61, Bl59, GB29, SI10, Co15, Co16, St4, St3, St1, Bl1, GB20 (Lo pt Bl62)	Bl62
Dai Mai	Li13, GB26, GB27, GB28 (Lo pt GB28)	GB41
Yang Wei Mai	Bl63, GB35, SI10, TH15, GB21, St8, GB13, GB14, GB15, GB16, GB17, GB18, GB19, GB20, GV16, GV15 (Lo pt Bl63)	TH5
Ren Mai	Own specific points (Lo pt CV15)	Lu7
Yin Chiao Mai	Ki2, Ki6, Ki8, Bl1 (Lo pt Ki6)	Ki6
Chong Mai	St30, Ki11 to Ki21 inclusive (Lo pt Ki11)	Sp4
Yin Wei Mai	Ki9, Sp13, Sp15, Sp16, Li14, CV22, CV23 (Lo pt Ki9)	HC6

Eight Influential Points

Tsang Organs	Li13
Fu Organs	CV12
Ch'i (& Respiratory)	CV17
Blood	Bl17
Vessels & Pulse	Lu9
Tendons	GB34
Bone	Bl11
Marrow	GB39

The 'Four Seas'

Sea of Energy	CV17, St9, Bl10
Sea of Nourishment	St30, St36
Sea of Meridians	Bl11, St37, St39
Sea of Marrow	GV16, GV20 (Query GV17)

'Windows of the Sky'

St9, Co18, TH16, Bl10, Lu3
(Secondary pts: GV15, CV22, SI16, SI17, HC1)

The Six Chiaos

		Root	*Concentration*
Tai Yang (Great Yang)	Bl/SI	Bl67	Bl1
Shao Yang (Lesser Yang)	GB/TH	GB44	GB3
Yang Ming (Bright Yang)	St/Co	St45	St3
Tai Yin (Great Yin)	Sp/Lu	Sp1	CV12
Chueh Yin (Absolute Yin)	Li/HC	Li1	CV18
Shao Yin (Lesser Yin)	Ki/Ht	Ki1	CV23

Lower Ho Points

St	St36
Co	St37
SI	St39
GB	GB34
Bl	Bl54
TH	Bl53

Group Lo Points

TH8 — controls SI, Co, TH (Upper Yang)
HC5 — controls Lu, HC, Ht (Upper Yin)
GB39 — controls GB, St, Bl (Lower Yang)
Sp6 — controls Sp, Li, Ki (Lower Yin)

The Five-Transformation Correspondences

Element	WOOD	FIRE	EARTH	METAL	WATER
Direction	East	South	Centre	West	North
Colour	Green	Red	Yellow	White	Black
Season	Spring	Summer	Long Summer	Autumn	Winter
Climate	Wind	Heat	Humidity	Dryness	Cold
Process	Birth	Growth	Transformation (Maturity)	Harvest	Storage
Nourishes	Muscles	Blood Vessels	Flesh	Skin	Bones
Expands into	Nails	Colour	Lips	Body Hair	Head Hair
Orifice	Eyes	Tongue	Mouth	Nose	Ears
Sense	Sight	Speech	Taste	Smell	Hearing
Flavour	Sour	Bitter	Sweet	Pungent	Salt
Body Smell	Rancid	Scorched	Fragrant	Rank	Putrid
Liquid emitted	Tears	Sweat	Saliva	Mucus	Urine
Emotion	Aggression	Joy	Calmness	Sympathy	Caution
Excess Emotion	Anger	Over-Excitement	Depression	Grief	Fear
Human Sound	Shout	Laughter	Singing	Weeping	Groaning
Chinese Note	Chio	Chih	Kung	Shang	Yu
Meat	Chicken	Mutton	Beef	Horse	Pork
Cereal	Wheat	Rice	Maize	Oats	Beans

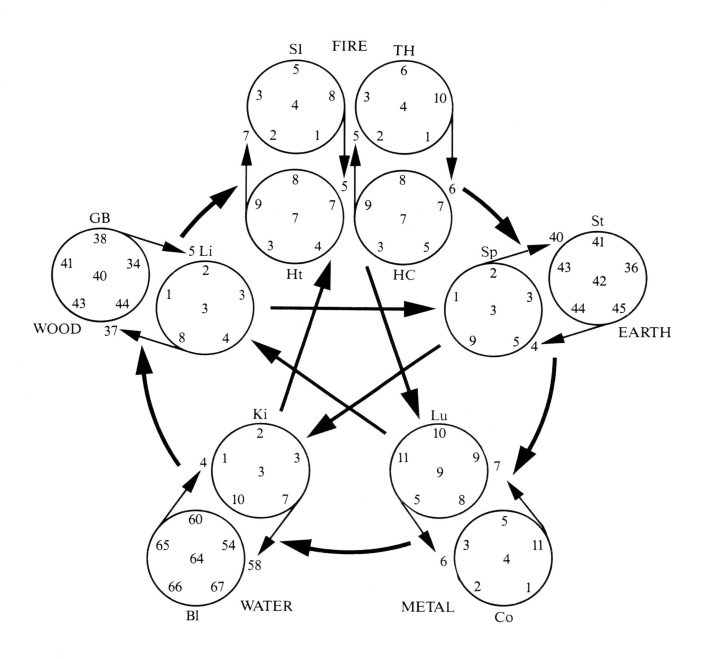

THE FIVE TRANSFORMATIONS

The Chinese Clock

Meridian	Hours	Horary Point
Lu	03-05	Lu8
Co	05-07	Co1
St	07-09	St36
Sp	09-11	Sp3
Ht	11-13	Ht8
SI	13-15	SI5
Bl	15-17	Bl66
Ki	17-19	Ki10
HC	19-21	HC8
TH	21-23	TH6
GB	23-01	GB41
Li	01-03	Li1

Law of Mid-Day/Mid-Night:

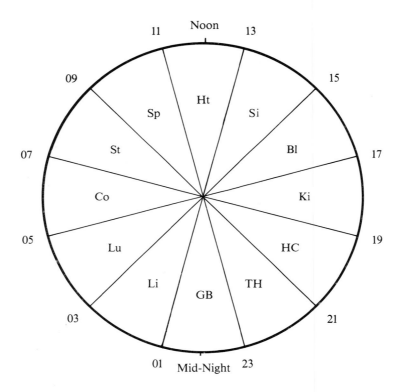

'An action taken on one organ will have an opposite action on the organ diametrically opposite it'. The action is strongest if a Yin organ is stimulated in a Yin time (12-24 hours) and a Yang organ in a Yang time (24-12 hours).

In practice it is found that only strong stimulation calls the Law into effect — if an organ is given only moderate stimulation, then that organ alone is affected. Also in practice, the energies do tend to equalize themselves, i.e. by tonifying the Sp in the afternoon the TH would be sedated, but if the TH were already in a depleted state, then tonification of the Sp would tend to reinforce it and bring both Sp and TH to a more balanced condition.

INDEX OF POINTS IN PINYIN

Guanyuanshu	Bl26	Kongzui	Lu6	Qingling	Ht2
Guilai	St29	Kufang	St14	Qishe	St11
		Kunlun	Bl60	Qiuxu	GB40
Hanyan	GB4			Qixue	Ki13
Hegu	Co4	Laogong	HC8	Quanliao	SI18
Heliao (Ear)	TH22	Liangmen	St21	Qubin	GB7
Heliao (Nose)	Co19	Liangqui	St34	Quchai	Bl4
Henggu	Ki11	Lianquan	CV23	Quchi	Co11
Heyang	Bl55	Lidui	St45	Quepen	St12
Houding	GV19	Lieque	Lu7	Qugu	CV2
Houxi	SI3	Ligou	Li5	Ququan	Li8
Huagai	CV20	Lingdao	Ht4	Quze	HC3
Huangmen	Bl46	Lingtai	GV10		
Huangshu	Ki16	Lingxu	Ki24	Rangu	Ki2
Huantiao	GB30	Linqi (Foot)	GB41	Renying	St9
Huaroumen	St24	Linqi (Head)	GB15	Renzhong	GV26
Huiyang	Bl35	Lougu	Sp7	Riyue	GB24
Huiyin	CV1	Luoque	Bl8	Rugen	St18
Huizong	TH7	Luxi	TH19	Ruzhong	St17
Hunmen	Bl42				
		Meichong	Bl3	Sanjian	Co3
Jiache	St6	Mingmen	GV4	Sanjiaoshu	Bl22
Jianjing	GB21	Muchuang	GB16	Sanyangluo	TH8
Jianli	CV11			Sanyinjiao	Sp6
Jianliao	TH14	Nauhu	GV17	Shangguan	GB3
Jianshi	HC5	Naohui	TH13	Shangjuxu	St37
Jianwaishu	SI14	Naokong	GB19	Shanglian	Co9
Jianyu	Co15	Naoshu	SI10	Shangliao	Bl31
Jianzhen	SI9	Neiguan	HC6	Shangqiu	Sp5
Jianzhongshu	SI15	Neiting	St44	Shangqu	Ki17
Jiaosun	TH20			Shangwan	CV13
Jiaoxin	Ki8	Pangguangshu	Bl28	Shangxing	GV23
Jiexi	St41	Pianli	Co6	Shangyang	Co1
Jimai	Li12	Pishu	Bl20	Shanzhong	CV17
Jimen	Sp11	Pohu	Bl37	Shaochong	Ht9
Jinggu	Bl64	Pushen	Bl61	Shaofu	Ht8
Jingmen	GB25			Shaohai	Ht3
Jingming	Bl1	Qianding	GV21	Shaoshang	Lu11
Jingqu	Lu8	Qiangjian	GV18	Shaoze	SI1
Jinmen	Bl63	Qiangu	SI2	Shencang	Ki25
Jinsuo	GV8	Qiaoyin (Foot)	GB44	Shendao	GV11
Jiquan	Ht1	Qiaoyin (Head)	GB11	Shenfeng	Ki23
Jiuwei	CV15	Qichong	St30	Shenmai	Bl62
Jizhong	GV6	Qihai	CV6	Shenmen	Ht7
Jueyinshu	Bl14	Qihaishu	Bl24	Shenque	CV8
Jugu	Co16	Qihu	St13	Shenshu	Bl23
Juliao (Leg)	GB29	Qimai	TH18	Shentang	Bl39
Juliao (Face)	St3	Qimen	Li14	Shenting	GV24
Juque	CV14	Qinglengyuan	TH11	Shenzhu	GV12

Shidou	Sp17	Wailing	St26	Yangxi	Co5		
Shiguan	Ki18	Waiqiu	GB36	Yaoshu	GV2		
Shimen	CV5	Wangu (Hand)	SI4	Yaoyangguan	GV3		
Shousanli	Co10	Wangu (Head)	GB12	Yemen	TH2		
Shuaigu	GB8	Weicang	Bl45	Yifeng	TH17		
Shufu	Ki27	Weidao	GB28	Yinbai	Sp1		
Shugu	Bl65	Weishu	Bl21	Yinbao	Li9		
Shuidao	St28	Weiyang	Bl53	Yindu	Ki19		
Shuifen	CV9	Weizhong	Bl54	Yingchuang	St16		
Shuiquan	Ki5	Wenliu	Co7	Yingu	Ki10		
Shuitu	St10	Wuchu	Bl5	Yingxiang	Co20		
Sibai	St2	Wuli	Co13	Yinjiao (Abdomen)	CV7		
Sidu	TH9	Wushu	GB27	Yinjiao (Mouth)	GV28		
Siman	Ki14	Wuyi	St15	Yinlian	Li11		
Sizhukong	TH23			Yinlingquan	Sp9		
Suliao	GV25	Xiabai	Lu4	Yinmen	Bl51		
		Xiaguan	St7	Yinshi	St33		
Taibai	Sp3	Xiajuxu	St39	Yinxi	Ht6		
Taichong	Li3	Xialian	Co8	Yishe	Bl44		
Taixi	Ki3	Xialiao	Bl34	Yixi	Bl39		
Taiyi	St23	Xiangu	St43	Yongquan	Ki1		
Taiyuan	Lu9	Xiaochangshu	Bl27	Youmen	Ki21		
Taodao	GV13	Xiaohai	SI8	Yuanye	GB22		
Tianchi	HC1	Xiaoluo	TH12	Yuji	Lu10		
Tianchong	GB9	Xiawan	CV10	Yunmen	Lu2		
Tianchuang	SI16	Xiaxi	GB43	Yutang	CV18		
Tianding	Co17	Xiguan	Li7	Yuzhen	Bl9		
Tianfu	Lu3	Ximen	HC4	Yuzhong	Ki26		
Tianjing	TH10	Xingjian	Li2				
Tianliao	TH15	Xinhui	GV22	Zanzhu	Bl2		
Tianquan	HC2	Xinshu	Bl15	Zhangmen	Li13		
Tianrong	SI17	Xiongxiang	Sp19	Zhaohai	Ki6		
Tianshu	St25	Xiyangguan	GB33	Zhejin	GB23		
Tiantu	CV22	Xuanji	CV21	Zhengying	GB17		
Tianxi	Sp18	Xuanli	GB6	Zhibian	Bl49		
Tianyou	TH16	Xuanlu	GB5	Zhigou	TH6		
Tianzhu	Bl10	Xuanshu	GV5	Zhishi	Bl47		
Tianzong	SI11	Xuanzhong	GB39	Zhiyang	GV9		
Tiaokou	St38	Xuehai	Sp10	Zhiyin	Bl67		
Tinggong	SI19			Zhizheng	SI7		
Tinghui	GB2	Yamen	GV15	Zhongchong	HC9		
Tonggu (Abdomen)	Ki20	Yangbai	GB14	Zhongdu (Leg)	GB32		
Tonggu (Foot)	Bl66	Yangchi	TH4	Zhongdu (Foot)	Li6		
Tongli	Ht5	Yangfu	GB38	Zhongfeng	Li4		
Tongtian	Bl7	Yanggang	Bl43	Zhongfu	Lu1		
Tongziliao	GB1	Yanggu	SI5	Zhongji	CV3		
Touwei	St8	Yangjiao	GB35	Zhongliao	Bl33		
		Yanglao	SI6	Zhonglüshu	Bl29		
Waiguan	TH5	Yanglingquan	GB34	Zhongshu	GV7		

Zhongting	CV16	Zhongzhu (Hand)	TH3	Zhubin	Ki9
Zhongwan	CV12	Zhouliao	Co12	Zigong	CV19
Zhongzhu (Abdomen)	Ki15	Zhourong	Sp20	Zusanli	St36

INDEX OF POINTS IN WADE-GILES

Changchiang	GV1	Chienli	CV11	Chingmen	GB25
Changmen	Li13	Chienliao	TH14	Chingming	Bl1
Chaohai	Ki6	Chienshih	HC5	Chinmen	Bl63
Chechin	GB23	Chienting	GV21	Chinso	GV8
Chengchi	St1	Chienwaishu	SI14	Chishe	St11
Changchiang	CV24	Chienyu	Co15	Chiuhsu	GB40
Changchin	Bl56	Chihai	CV6	Chiuwei	CV15
Chengfu	Bl50	Chihaishu	Bl24	Choujung	Sp20
Chengkuang	Bl6	Chihcheng	SI7	Chouliao	Co12
Chengling	GB18	Chihkou	TH6	Chuanliao	SI18
Chengman	St20	Chihmo	TH18	Chucha	Bl4
Chengshan	Bl57	Chihpien	Bl49	Chuchih	Co11
Chengying	GB17	Chihshih	Bl47	Chuchuan	Li8
Chiache	St6	Chihsueh	Ki13	Chuchueh	CV14
Chiangchien	GV18	Chihtse	Lu5	Chuehpen	St12
Chiaohsin	Ki8	Chihu	St13	Chuehsun	TH20
Chiaoyin	GB11	Chihyang	GV9	Chuehyinshu	Bl14
Chich'uan	Ht1	Chiyin	Bl67	Chuku (Arm)	Co16
Chichung	GV6	Chimen	Sp11	Chuku (Trunk)	CV2
Ch'ich'ung	St30	Ch'imen	Ki14	Chuliao (Trunk)	GB29
Chiehhsi	St41	Chimo	Li12	Chuliao (Face)	St3
Chiencheng	SI9	Chingchu	Lu8	Chungchi	CV3
Chienching	GB21	Chingku	Bl64	Chungchu (Hand)	TH3
Chienchungshu	SI15	Chinglengyuan	TH11	Chungchu (Trunk)	Ki15
Chienku	SI2	Ch'ingling	Ht2	Chungchung	HC9

Chungfeng	Li4	Hsialien	Co8	Kungtsui	Lu6
Chungfu	Lu1	Hsiawan	CV10	Kunlun	Bl60
Chungliao	Bl33	Hsiaochangshu	Bl27		
Chunglushu	Bl29	Hsiaohai	SI8	Laokung	HC8
Chungmen	Sp12	Hsiaolo	TH12	Liangchiu	St34
Chungshu	GV7	Hsiapai	Lu4	Liangmen	St21
Chungting	CV16	Hsienku	St43	Liehchueh	Lu7
Chungtu (GB)	GB32	Hsikuan	Li7	Lienchuan	CV23
Chungtu (Li)	Li6	Hsimen	HC4	Likou	Li5
Chungwan	CV12	Hsingchien	Li2	Linchi	GB15
Chungyang	St42	Hsinshu	Bl15	Linghsu	Ki24
Chupin	Ki9	Hsinhui	GV22	Lingtai	GV10
Ch'upin	GB7	Hsiunghsiang	Sp19	Lingtao	Ht4
Chutse	HC3	Hsiyangkuan	GB33	Litui	St45
Chuyuan	SI13	Hsuanchi	CV21	Lochueh	Bl8
		Hsuanchung	GB39	Louku	Sp7
Erhchien	Co2	Hsuanli	GB6	Luhsi	TH19
Erhmen	TH21	Hsuanlu	GB5		
		Hsuanshu	GV5	Meichung	Bl3
Feishu	Bl13	Hsuehhai	Sp10	Mingmen	GV4
Feiyang	Bl58	Huajoumen	St24	Muchuang	GB16
Fengchih	GB20	Huakai	CV20		
Fengfu	GV16	Huangmen	Bl46	Naohu	GV17
Fenglung	St40	Huangshu	Ki16	Naohui	TH13
Fengmen	Bl12	Huantiao	GB30	Naokung	GB19
Fengshih	GB31	Huitsung	TH7	Naoshu	SI10
Fuai	Sp16	Huiyang	Bl35	Neikuan	HC6
Fuchieh	Sp14	Huijin	CV1	Neiting	St44
Fufen	Bl36	Hunmen	Bl42		
Fuhsi	Bl52			Paihuanshu	Bl30
Fuliu	Ki7	Janku	Ki2	Paihui	GV20
Fupai	GB10	Jenchung	GV26	Pangkuangshu	Bl28
Fushe	Sp13	Jenying	St9	Paohuang	Bl48
Futu (St)	St32	Jihyueh	GB24	Penshen	GB13
Futu (Co)	Co18	Juchung	St17	Pienli	Co6
Fuyang	Bl59	Juken	St18	Pikuan	St31
				Pinao	Co14
Hanyen	GB4	Kanshu	Bl18	Pingfeng	SI12
Hengku	Ki11	Kaohuang	Bl38	Pishu	Bl20
Hoku	Co4	Kekuan	Bl41	Pohu	Bl37
Holiao (Co)	Co19	Keshu	Bl17	Pujung	St19
Holiao (TH)	TH22	Kuanchung	TH1	Pulang	Ki22
Houhsi	SI3	Kuangming	GB37	Pushen	Bl61
Houting	GV19	Kuanmen	St22		
Hoyang	Bl55	Kuanyuan	CV4	Sanchiaoshu	Bl22
Hsiachuhsu	St39	Kuanyuanshu	Bl26	Sanchien	Co3
Hsiahsi	GB43	Kufang	St14	Sanli	Co10
Hsiakuan	St7	Kuilai	St29	Sanyanglo	TH8
Hsialiao	Bl34	Kungsun	Sp4	Sanyinchiao	Sp6

Shanchung	CV17	Taihsi	Ki3	Waichiu	GB36
Shangchui	Sp5	Taimo	GB26	Waikuan	TH5
Shangchu	Ki17	Taipai	Sp3	Wailing	St26
Shangchuhsu	St37	Taiyi	St23	Wanku (GB)	GB12
Shanghsing	GV23	Taiyuan	Lu9	Wanku (Si)	SI4
Shangkuan	GB3	Taling	HC7	Weichung	Bl54
Shangliao	Bl31	Tanshu	Bl19	Weishu	Bl21
Shanglien	Co9	Taotao	GV13	Weitao	GB28
Shangwan	CV13	Tapao	Sp21	Weitsang	Bl45
Shangyang	Co1	Tatu	Sp2	Weiyang	Bl53
Shaochung	Ht9	Tatun	Li1	Wenliu	Co7
Shaofu	Ht8	Taying	St5	Wuchu	Bl5
Shaohai	Ht3	Tiaokou	St38	Wuli (Thigh)	Li10
Shaoshang	Lu11	Tichi	Sp8	Wuli (Arm)	Co13
Shaotse	SI1	Tienchih	HC1	Wushu	GB27
Shenchu	GV12	Tienching	TH10	Wuyi	St15
Shenchueh	CV8	Tienchu	Bl10		
Shenfeng	Ki23	Tienchung	GB9	Yamen	GV15
Shenmen	Ht7	Tienchuan	HC2	Yangchiao	GB35
Shenmo	Bl62	Tienchuang	SI16	Yangchih	TH4
Shenshu	Bl23	Tienfu	Lu3	Yangfu	GB38
Shentang	Bl39	Tienhsi	Sp18	Yanghsi	Co5
Shentao	GV11	Tienjung	SI17	Yangkang	Bl43
Shenting	GV24	Tienliao	TH15	Yangku	SI5
Shentsang	Ki25	Tienshu	St25	Yangkuan	GV3
Shihkuan	Ki18	Tienting	Co17	Yanglao	SI6
Shihmen	CV5	Tientsung	SI11	Yanglingchuan	GB34
Shihtou	Sp17	Tientu	CV22	Yangpai	GB14
Shuaiku	GB8	Tienyu	TH16	Yaoshu	GV2
Shufu	Ki27	Tinghui	GB2	Yemen	TH2
Shuichuan	Ki5	Tingkung	SI19	Yifeng	TH17
Shuifen	CV9	Titsang	St4	Yihsi	Bl40
Shuitao	St28	Tiwuhui	GB42	Yinchiao (Jen Mo)	CV7
Shuitu	St10	Touwei	St8	Yinchiao (Tu Mo)	GV28
Shuku	Bl65	Tsanchu	Bl2	Yingchuang	St16
Ssuchukung	TH23	Tsuchiaoyin	GB44	Yinghsiang	Co20
Suliao	GV25	Tsulinchi	GB41	Yinhsi	Ht6
Szuman	Ki14	Tsusanli	St36	Yinku	Ki10
Szupai	St2	Tuituan	GB27	Yinlien	Li11
Szutu	TH9	Tungku (Bl)	Bl66	Yinlingchuan	Sp9
		Tungku (Ki)	Ki20	Yinmen	Bl51
Tachangshu	Bl25	Tungli	Ht5	Yinpai	Sp1
Tachui	GV14	Tungtien	Bl7	Yinpao	Li9
Tachu	Bl11	Tungtzuliao	GB1	Yinshih	St33
Tachü	St27	Tupi	St35	Yintu	Ki19
Tachung	Ki4	Tushu	Bl16	Yishe	Bl44
Taheh	Ki12	Tzukung	CV19	Yuanyeh	GB22
Taheng	Sp15	Tzuliao	Bl32	Yuchen	Bl9
Taichung	Li3			Yuchi	Lu10

| Yuchung | Ki26 | Yungchuan | Ki1 | Yutang | CV18 |
| Yumen | Ki21 | Yunmen | Lu2 | | |